Hospital Safety
FOR KIDS

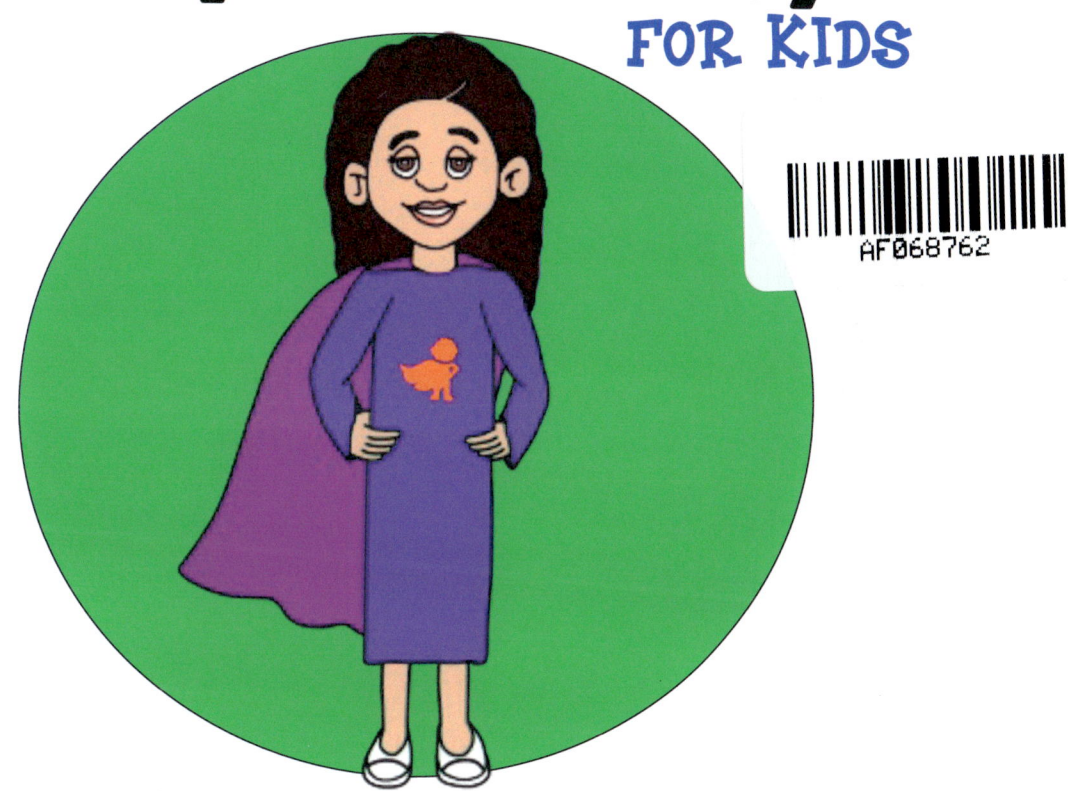

by Charisse N. Montgomery • illustrated by Davina Westbrook

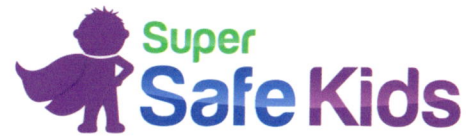

For the LITTLE BUG and the BUTTERFLY

Special thanks to the Patient and Family Partnership Council at University Hospitals Rainbow Babies & Children's Hospital, Cleveland, Ohio

© 2017 Black and Blue Publishing. All rights reserved. No part of this publication may be reproduced or transmitted in any form or by any means, electronic or mechanical, including photography, recording, or any information storage or retrieval system, without permission in writing from the publisher. Printed in the United States. For ordering information, visit our website at www.supersafekidsbooks.com.

ISBN: 978-0-9861761-7-3

Hospital Safety FOR KIDS

How to use this book with children:

- Read the book aloud regularly with the child and siblings, friends or classmates.
- Talk about what it means to be part of the health care team.
- Talk about why it is important to tell hospital staff how you are feeling.
- Talk about why it is important to listen to doctors and nurses without being distracted.
- Bring this book for hospital stays and visits, and practice the skills in the book.

Concepts and words used in this book:

Safety	Germs and hand washing
Health care team	Advocacy
Wellness	Listening and asking questions

A health care team is made up of all the people who work hard to make sure I stay healthy.

When I'm in the hospital, my family and I are part of the health care team.

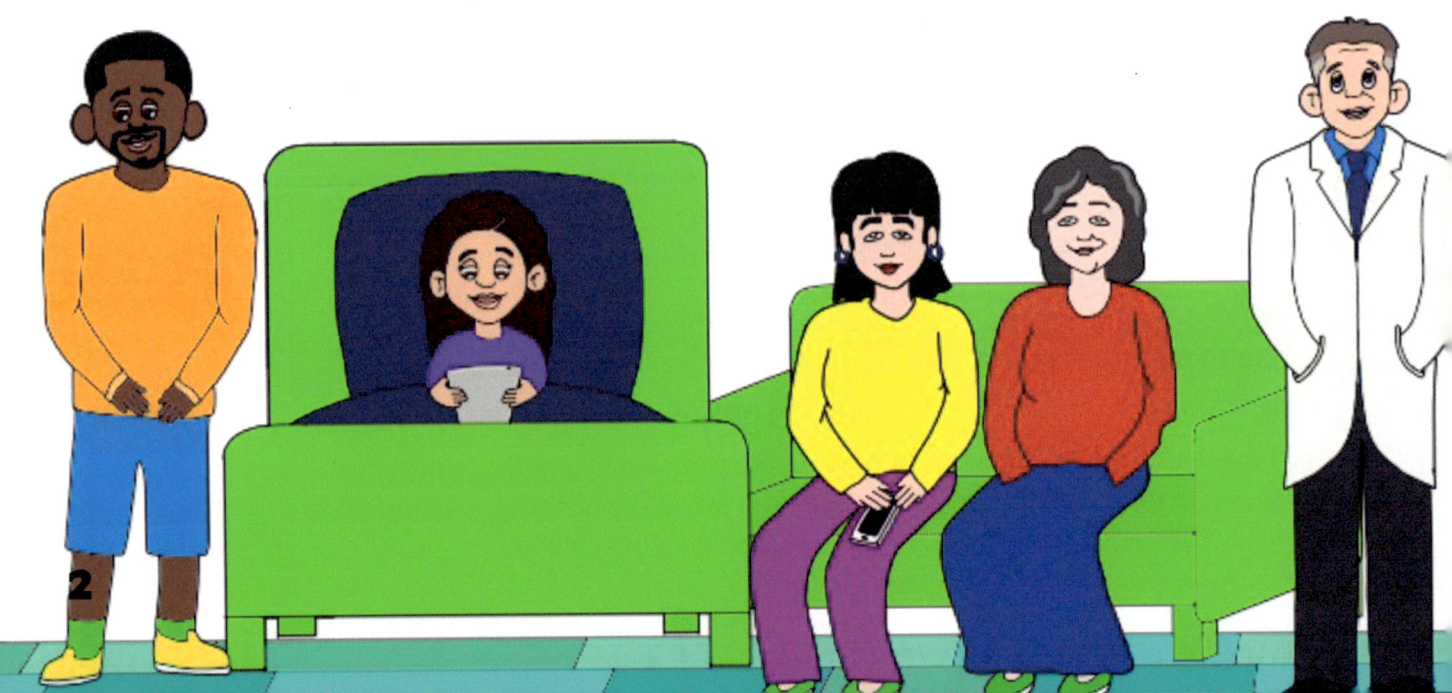

The doctors and nurses listen to me and my family, and we all work together
to keep me healthy and safe.

They explain things to us and
make sure we understand.

We put away our phones, tablets and computers
so we can listen carefully to the
nurses, doctors and other hospital workers.

Staying well is very important
to my family and me,
so we learn all we can about what is
happening while I'm in the hospital
and talk about our concerns.

We ask questions and write notes
about what we learn.

If I have a question and a nurse is not nearby, my family writes my question in a notebook so I can ask it later.

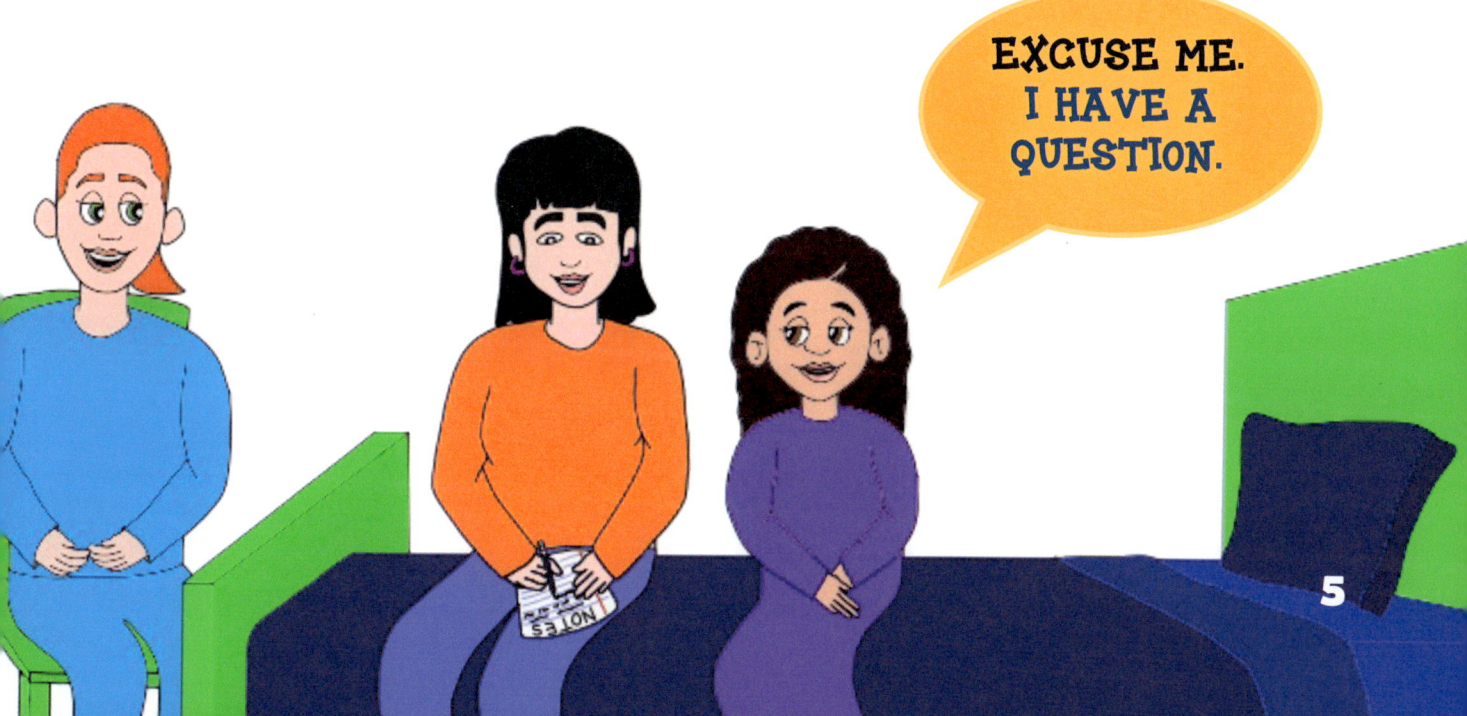

When hospital workers visit my room,
I like to find out what they do
and how they will help me.

HELLO!
WHAT IS YOUR NAME?
WHAT DO YOU DO HERE?

I learn the names of the people who are helping to take care of me, and I tell them how I'm feeling and what I need.

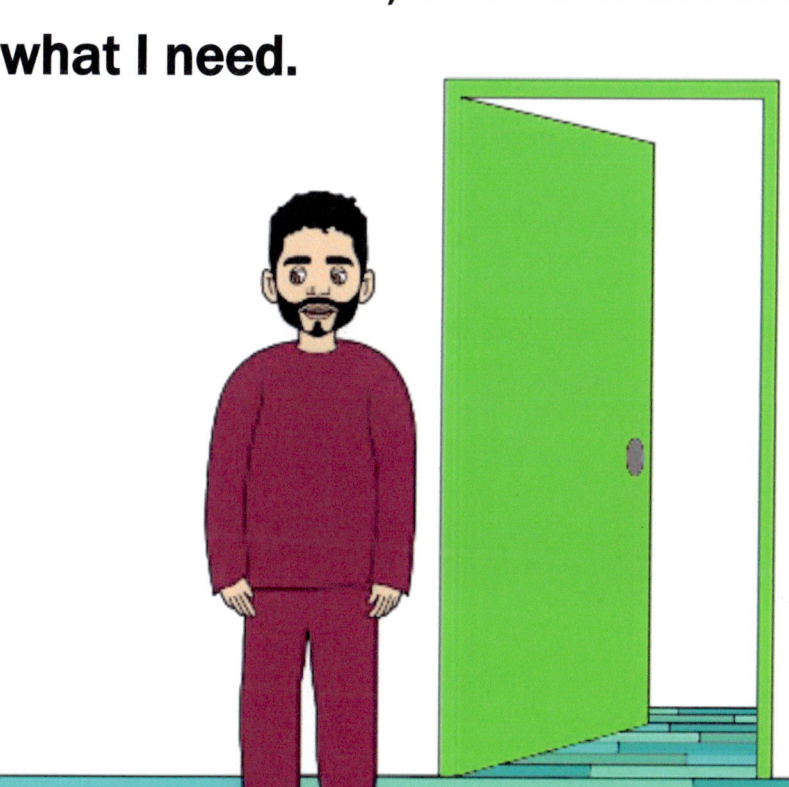

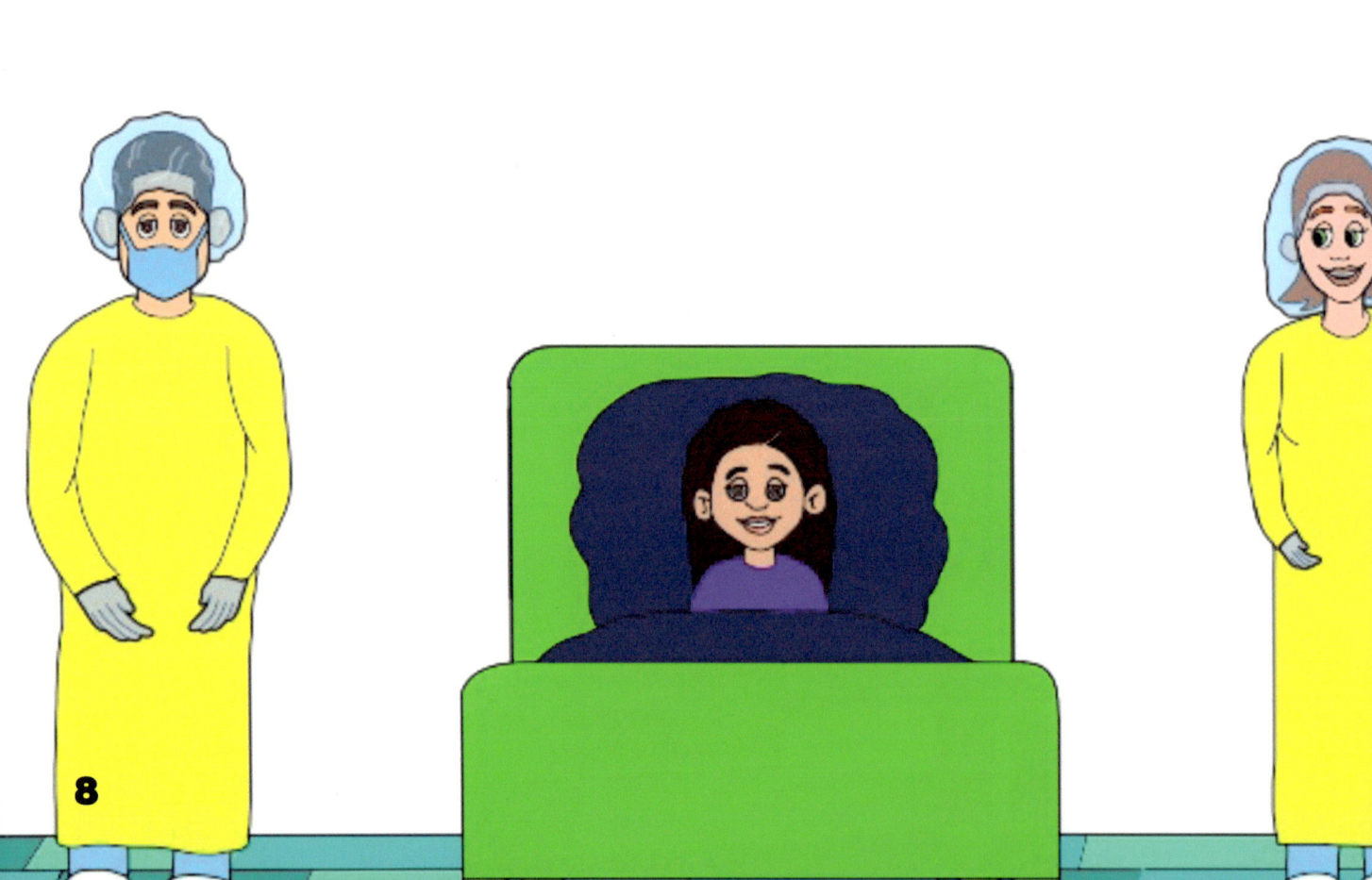

The doctors and nurses might wear special clothes
like gloves, masks and gowns
when they come into my hospital room.

Everyone who comes to my room
has to wash their hands.
I watch to make sure that
all hands in the room are clean.

This keeps germs away,
which can help me to feel better.

When I'm in the hospital, I can go to rounds.
Rounds are when my family, my nurse
and all my doctors talk about my care
and think about how to help me feel better.

I follow the hospital's safety rules
and remind my family and visitors to follow them, too.
The rules help everyone stay safe in the hospital.

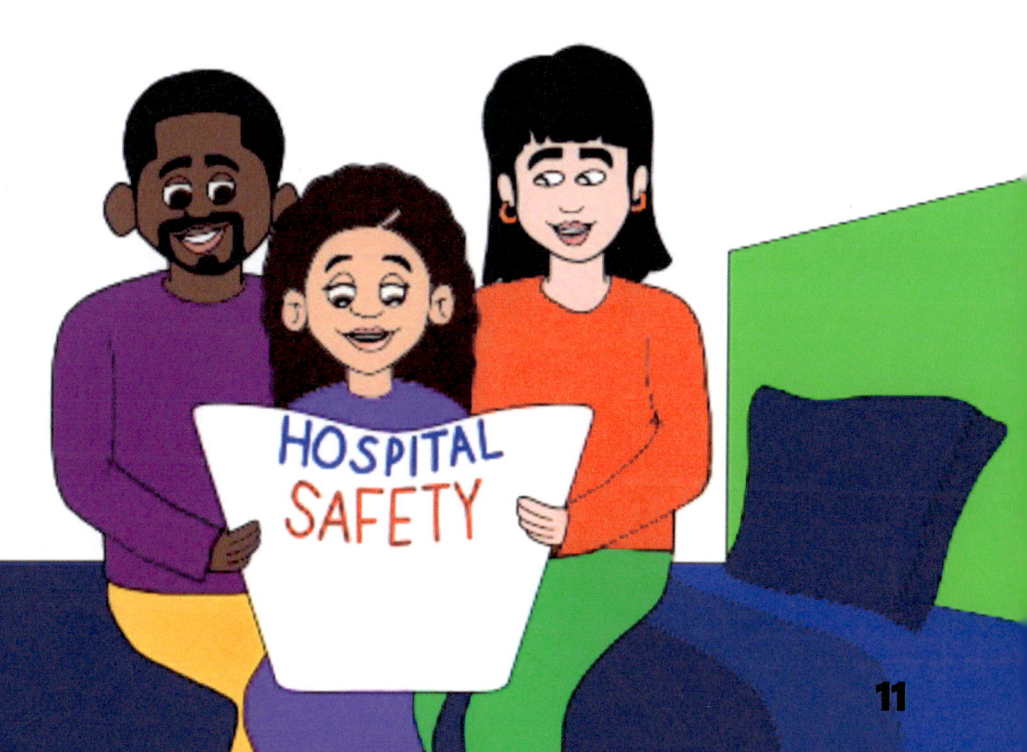

My family and I learn about the medication I'm taking in the hospital.

We write down the name of each medication,
why I'm taking it,
the dose and time I take it,
and how it might make me feel.

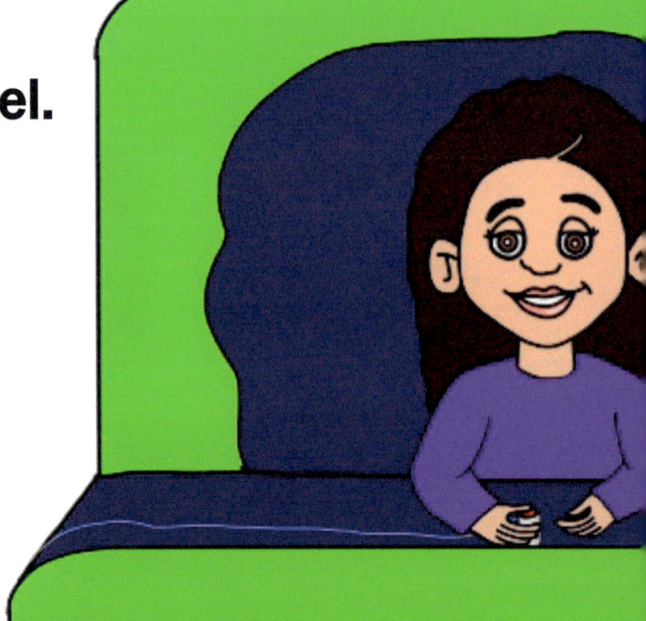

When my body hurts or
when I need to move around,
I ask someone to help me.

I can press the call button in my room
when I need help.

If I start feeling different or feeling worse,
I tell my family and the other members
of my health care team.

When it's time to go home, I listen
so I know what I have to do
at home to stay healthy.

My family and I make plans to
get any medications I will need at home.

We also make an appointment
to see my doctor later.

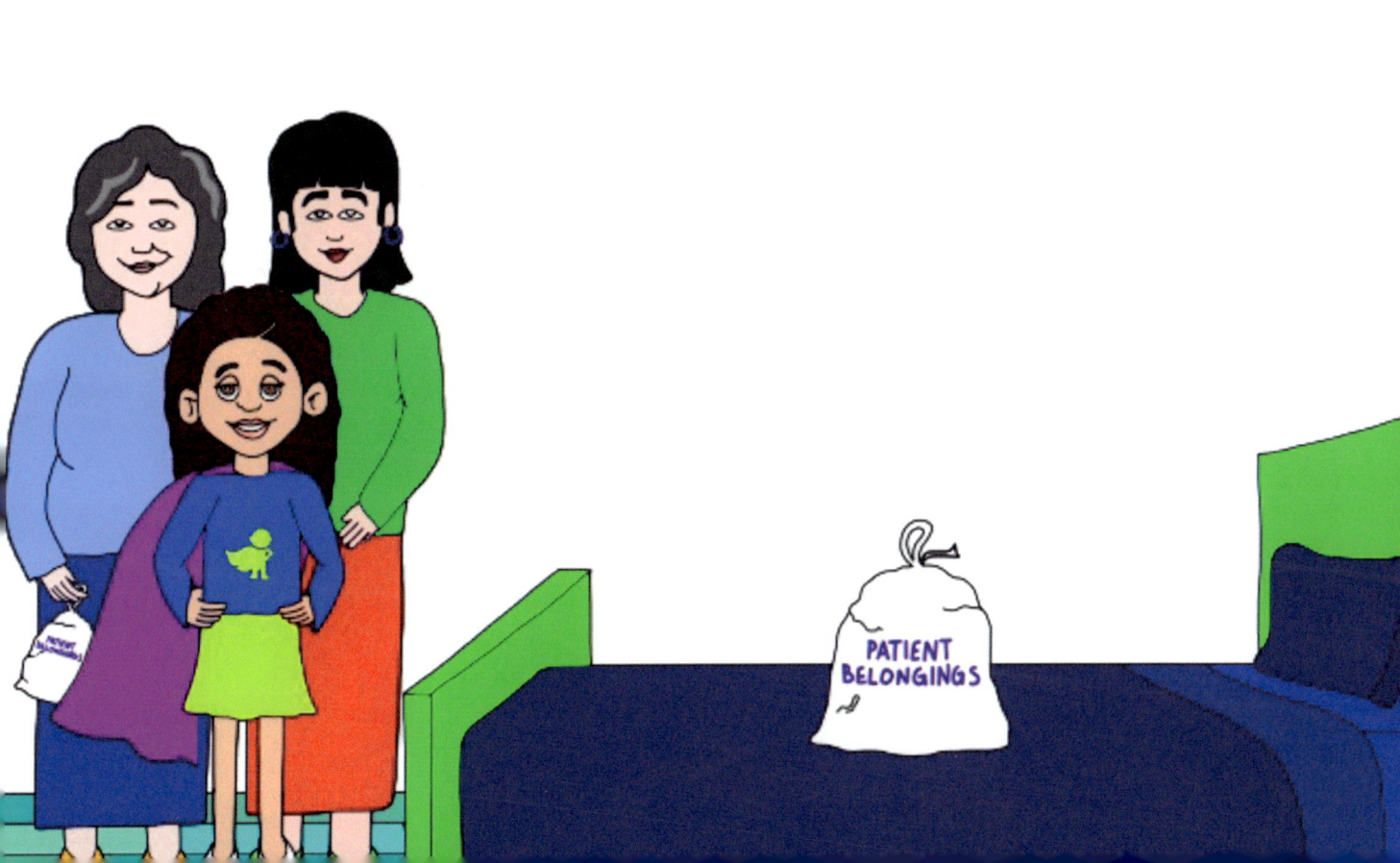

I listen, learn and speak up for safety when I'm at the hospital.
My family does, too!

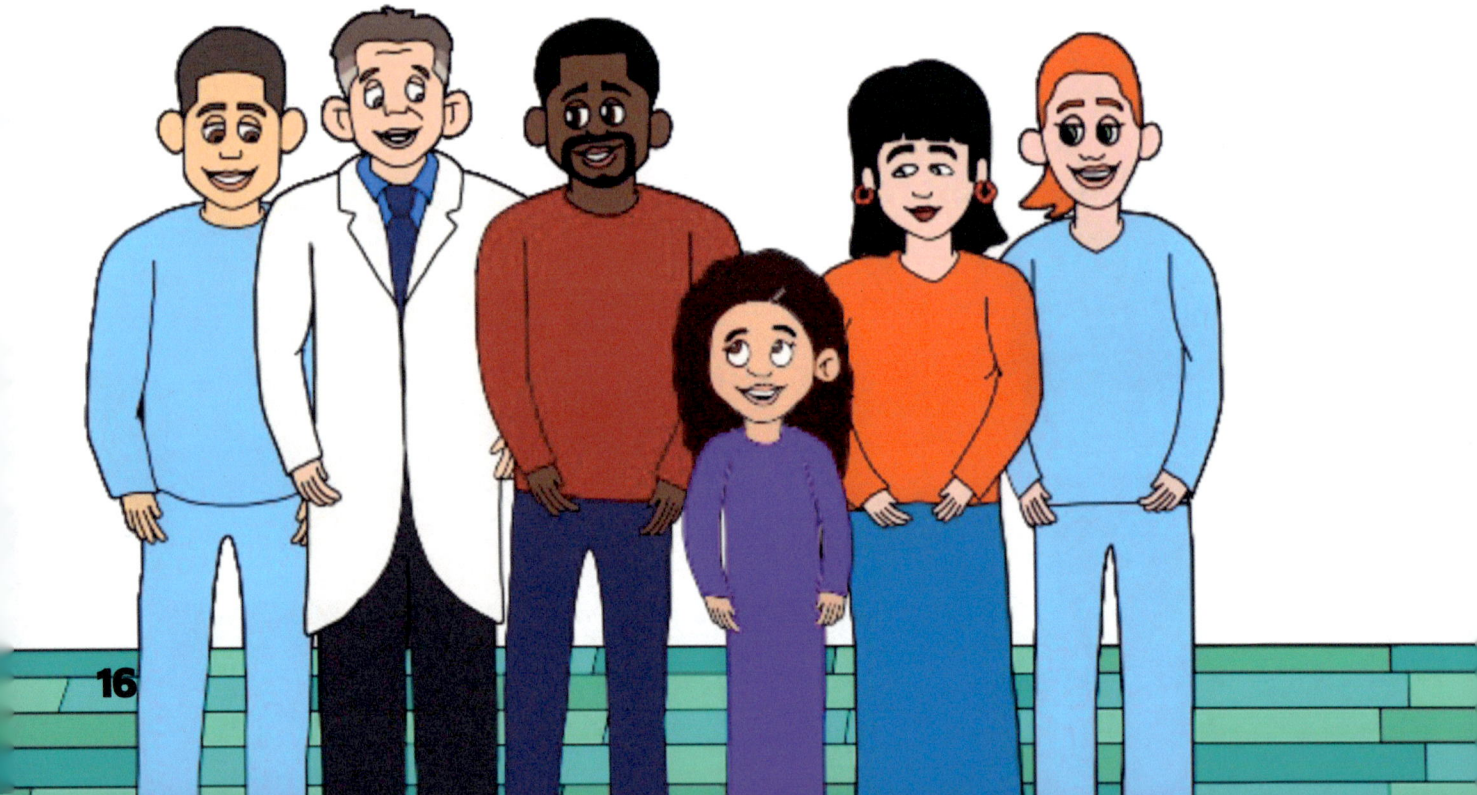

I'm part of the
health care team,
and I'm a Super Safe Kid.

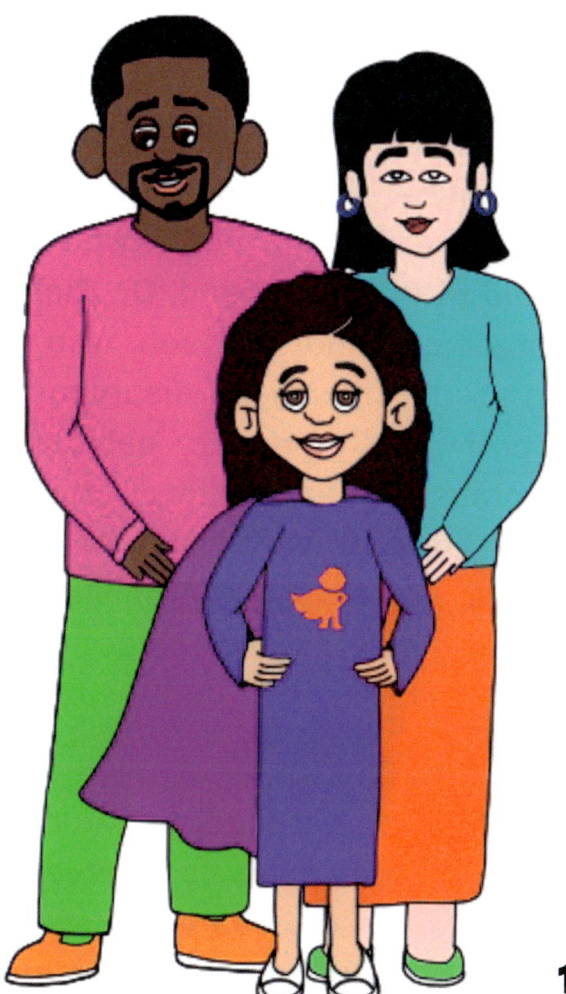

About the Author, Charisse N. Montgomery, M.A., M.Ed., GPAC

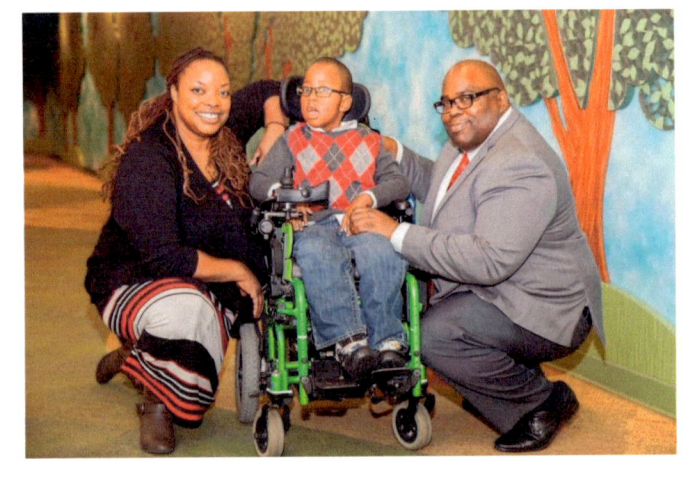

Charisse Montgomery is the author of the Super Safe Kids book series. She is a writer and editor who lives in Ohio with her husband, Dr. Richard Montgomery, and their son, who was born with fiber-type disproportion myopathy, a rare and debilitating neuromuscular condition. Charisse writes books that engage children, parents, and their families in improving safety and advocacy in the hospital, the community and the home.

A former educator, Charisse Montgomery has bachelor's and master's degrees in English, along with a master's degree in Educational Psychology, with research focused on informing and empowering parents of medically fragile children. She completed a graduate certificate in Patient Advocacy and serves on the board at University Hospitals Rainbow Babies & Children's Hospital, where she is president of the Patient and Family Partnership

Council. She was awarded the honorable mention for the 2016 Patients' View Impact Award, presented by the Patients' View Institute and The Leapfrog Group. Charisse is also a member of the editorial board for Pediatrics, the flagship journal of the American Academy of Pediatrics.

As a special education advocate, Charisse educates and engages teachers, therapists and parents of children with special education needs in the school setting. She has also served on her county's Board of Developmental Disabilities. Her writing can be found in Complex Child Magazine and The Mighty, in addition to a blog series called Teachable Moments that she wrote for ProMedica HealthConnect.

About the Illustrator, Davina Westbrook

Davina Westbrook, raised in Omaha, Nebraska, has been drawing since she was nine years old. Davina is a Scholastic Art and Writing Award Gold Key winner, and won with her piece entitled, "The Parlor." Davina is attending high school and looking forward to higher education with a major in sports nutrition.

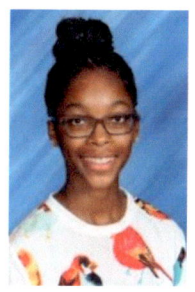

Follow Super Safe Kids books on Twitter @supersafekids

Join our Facebook page at Facebook.com/supersafekids

Visit our website at www.supersafekidsbooks.com

Made in the USA
Monee, IL
28 April 2026

49136492R00017